The Best Air Fryer Cooking Guide

Delicious Recipes to Stay Fit and Enjoy Your Air Fryer Diet

Franck McMillan

TABLE OF CONTENT

this book has been derived from various sources. Please consult a licensed professional before attempting any techniques outlined in this book.

By reading this document, the reader agrees that under no circumstances is the author responsible for any losses, direct or indirect, which are incurred as a result of the use of information contained within this document, including, but not limited to, — errors, omissions, or inaccuracies.

Pepper Feta Egg Muffins

Preparation Time:10 minutes

Cooking Time: 20 minutes

Servings:6

Ingredients:

- 4 eggs
- 1/2 cup egg whites
- red bell pepper, chopped
- tbsp green onion, chopped
- 5 fresh basil leaves, chopped
- tsp garlic powder
- tbsp feta cheese, crumbled
- 1/4 cup of coconut milk

Directions:

1. In a bowl, whisk eggs, egg whites, coconut milk, garlic powder, pepper, and salt.
2. Add cheese, bell pepper, green onion, and basil and stir well.
3. Pour egg mixture into the silicone muffin molds.
4. Place molds into the air fryer basket and cook at 350 F for 20 minutes.

Nutrition: Calories 92 Fat 6.1 g Carbohydrates 3.1 g

Sugar 2 g Protein 6.9 g Cholesterol 112 mg

Egg Bacon Muffins

Preparation Time:10 minutes

Cooking Time: 12 minutes

Servings:6

Ingredients:

- 4 eggs, lightly beaten
- 2 tbsp coconut milk
- 2 bacon slices, cooked and crumbled
- 2 tbsp cheddar cheese, shredded
- Pepper
- Salt

Directions:

1. In a bowl, whisk eggs with milk, pepper, and salt. Add bacon and cheese and stir well.
2. Pour egg mixture into the silicone muffin molds.
3. Place molds into the air fryer basket and cook at 350 F for 12 minutes.
4. Serve and enjoy.

Nutrition: Calories 97 Fat 7.5 g Carbohydrates 0.6 g Sugar 0.4 g Protein 6.7 g Cholesterol 119 mg

Greek Egg Muffins

Preparation Time:10 minutes

Cooking Time: 15 minutes

Servings:6

Ingredients:

- 2 eggs
- 1/4 cup tomatoes, diced
- 1/2 cup coconut milk
- 4 egg whites
- 1/4 cup feta cheese, crumbled
- tbsp fresh parsley, chopped
- 1/4 cup olives, diced
- 1/4 cup onion, diced
- Pepper
- Salt

Directions:

1. In a mixing bowl, whisk eggs with milk, pepper, and salt. Add remaining ingredients and stir well.
2. Pour egg mixture into the six silicone muffin molds.
3. Place molds into the air fryer basket and cook at 350 F for 15 minutes.

4. Serve and enjoy.

Nutrition: Calories 105 Fat 8.2 g Carbohydrates 2.8 g Sugar 1.6 g Protein 5.8 g Cholesterol 60 mg

Cheese Egg Breakfast Muffins

Preparation Time:10 minutes

Cooking Time: 5 minutes

Servings:4

Ingredients:

- 4 eggs
- 1/4 cup cheddar cheese, shredded
- 1/4 cup heavy cream
- Pepper
- Salt

Directions:

1. In a bowl, whisk eggs with heavy cream, cheese, pepper, and salt.
2. Pour egg mixture into the four silicone muffin molds.
3. Place muffin molds into the air fryer basket and cook at 350 F for 5 minutes.
4. Serve and enjoy.

Nutrition: Calories 117 Fat 9.5 g Carbohydrates 0.7 g Sugar 0.4 g Protein 7.5 g Cholesterol 181 mg

Cheese Sausage Egg Muffins

Preparation Time:10 minutes

Cooking Time: 5 minutes

Servings:6

Ingredients:

- 4 eggs
- 4 tbsp cheddar cheese, shredded
- 2 tbsp heavy cream
- 1/2 cup cooked sausage
- Pepper
- Salt

Directions:

1. Spray egg mold with cooking spray and set aside.
2. In a bowl, beat eggs until frothy. Add remaining Ingredients into the eggs and stir to mix.
3. Pour egg mixture into the egg mold.
4. Place egg mold into the air fryer basket and cook at 330 F for 5 minutes.
5. Serve and enjoy.

Nutrition: Calories 82 Fat 6.6 g Carbohydrates 0.4 g Sugar 0.3 g Protein 5.2 g Cholesterol 122 mg

Blueberry Cheese Muffins

Preparation Time:10 minutes

Cooking Time: 20 minutes

Servings:6

Ingredients:

- 8 oz cream cheese
- 1/4 tsp vanilla
- egg, lightly beaten
- 1/4 cup Swerve
- tbsp almonds, sliced
- tbsp blueberries

Directions:

1. Add the cream cheese in a mixing bowl and beat until smooth.
2. Add egg, vanilla, and sweetener and beat until well combined.
3. Add almonds and blueberries and fold well.
4. Spoon mixture into the silicone muffin molds.
5. Place molds into the air fryer basket and cook at 350 F for 20 minutes.
6. Serve and enjoy.

Nutrition: Calories 156, Fat 14.9g, Carbohydrates 2g,

Sugar 0.5g, Protein 4.2g, Cholesterol 69mg

Turkey Meatloaf Muffins

Preparation Time:10 minutes

Cooking Time: 35 minutes

Serves 12

Ingredients:

- ½ cup old-fashioned oats
- pound (454 g) lean ground turkey
- ½ cup finely chopped onion
- red bell pepper, seeded and finely chopped
- eggs
- garlic cloves, minced

Directions:

1. Preheat the oven to 375ºF (190ºC). Lightly spray a 12-cup muffin tin with nonstick cooking spray.
2. In a blender, process the oats until they become flour.
3. In a large mixing bowl, combine the oat flour, turkey, onion, bell pepper, eggs, and garlic. Mix well and season with the salt and pepper.

4. Using an ice cream scoop, transfer a ¼-cup portion of the meat mixture to each muffin cup.

5. Bake for 30 to 35 minutes until the muffins are cooked through.

6. Slide a knife along the outside of each cup to loosen the muffins and remove. Serve warm.

Nutrition: calories: 89 | fat: 4g | protein: 9g | carbs: 4g | sugars: 4g | fiber: 1g | sodium: 203mg

Corn, Orange, And Cranberry Muffins

Preparation and Cooking Time: 70 minutes

Servings: 15

Ingredients:

- cup cornmeal
- 0.75 cup flour
- teaspoon of baking powder
- 1 teaspoon of baking powder
- 1 teaspoon of salt
- 0.5 cup of sugar
- 4 tablespoons of butter
- 1 large egg
- 0.75 cup buttermilk
- 0.5 liquid pint us blueberries

Directions:

1. Mix cornmeal, flour, baking powder, baking powder, and salt in a bowl.
2. Mix the sugar and orange peel in a separate bowl and mix well to release the oils.
3. Add orange juice, butter, egg, and buttermilk to the sugar and the orange peel and whisk.

4. Combine the two bowls and add the blueberries to the mixture.

5. Pour the mixture into 15 foil cupcake liners. Place cupcake liners on two airflow racks. Arrange the racks on the button and middle shelves of the oven.

6. Press the power button (370 ° F for 15 minutes). Rotate the racks after 8 minutes.

7. Let the muffins cool and serve with butter.

Nutrition: Calories 90 Fat 6.4 g Carbohydrates 2 g Sugar 0.6 g Protein 6.5 g Cholesterol 129 mg

English Muffins

Preparation Time:3 Minutes

Cooking Time: 6 Minutes

Servings: 2

Ingredients:

- Two whole-wheat English muffins
- Four slices of bacon
- Pepper
- Two eggs

Directions:

1. Crack an egg each into ramekins, then season with pepper.
2. Place the ramekins in your preheated air fryer at 390 F.
3. Allow cooking for 6-minutes with the bacon and muffins alongside.
4. Remove the muffins from the air fryer after a few minutes and split them.
5. When the bacon and eggs are done cooking, add two bacon pieces and one egg to each egg muffin. Serve when hot.

Nutrition: Calories: 276 kcal Total Fat: 12g Carbs: 10.2g Protein: 17.3g

Cinnamon Muffins

Preparation Time:10 minutes

Cooking Time: 15 minutes

Servings:12

Ingredients:

- 4 eggs
- 1/2 cups almond flour
- 1tsp vanilla
- 1/4 cup unsweetened almond milk
- 2tbsp butter, melted
- 1/2 cup erythritol
- 1tsp psyllium husk
- 1/2 cup pecans, chopped
- 1/2 tsp ground cinnamon
- 2tsp allspice
- 1tbsp baking powder

Directions:

1. Preheat the air fryer to 400 F.
2. Beat eggs, milk, vanilla, sweetener, and butter in a bowl using a hand mixer until smooth.
3. Add remaining ingredients and stir until combined.

4. Pour batter into silicone muffin molds and
   place in the air fryer. In batches.

5. Cook for 15 minutes.

6. Serve and enjoy.

Nutrition: Calories 143 Fat 9 g Carbohydrates 8.1 g
Sugar 5.7 g Protein 9 g Cholesterol 175 mg

Easy Black and White Brownies

Preparation Time:10 minutes

Cooking Time: 20 minutes

Servings: 1 dozen brownies

Ingredients:

- egg
- 1/4cup brown sugar
- tablespoons white sugar
- tablespoons safflower oil
- 1 teaspoon vanilla
- 1/3cup all-purpose flour
- 1/4cup cocoa powder
- 1/4cup white chocolate chips
- Nonstick cooking spray

Directions:

1. Spritz a baking pan with nonstick cooking spray.

2. Whisk together the egg, white sugar, and brown sugar in a medium bowl. Mix in the vanilla and safflower oil and stir to combine.

3. Add the cocoa powder and flour and stir just until incorporated. Fold in the white chocolate chips.

4. Scrape the batter into the baking pan.

5. Place the pan on the bake position.

6. Select bake, set temperature to 340ºf (171ºc), and set Time to 20 minutes.

7. When done, the brownie should spring back when touched lightly with your fingers.

8. Transfer to a wire rack and let cool for 30 minutes before slicing to serve.

Nutrition: Calories 68 Fat 6.1 g Carbohydrates 1.2 g Sugar 0.3 g Protein 3 g Cholesterol 0 mg

Chocolate Brownie Bar

Preparation Time:10 minutes

Cooking Time: 16 minutes

Servings:4

Ingredients:

- cup bananas, overripe
- scoop protein powder
- tbsp unsweetened cocoa powder
- 1/2 cup almond butter, melted

Directions:

1. Preheat the air fryer to 325 f.
2. Spray air fryer baking pan with cooking spray.
3. Add all Ingredients into the blender and blend until smooth.
4. Pour batter into the pan and place in the air fryer basket.
5. Cook brownie for 16 minutes.
6. Serve and enjoy.

Nutrition: Calories: 164 Protein: 2 g. Fat: 22 g. Carbs: 4 g.

Brownies

Preparation Time:10 minutes

Cooking Time: 20 minutes

Servings: 2

Ingredients:

- ¼ cup of all-purpose flour
- ¼ teaspoon baking powder
- 1/3 cup of cocoa powder
- ¼ cup of butter
- ½ cup of granulated sugar
- egg, beaten Pinch salt

Directions:

1. Spray baking pan with oil.
2. In a bowl, mix all the ingredients.
3. Pour the mixture into the baking pan.
4. Set your air fryer to bake.
5. Cook at 350 degrees F for 18 to twenty minutes.
6. Serving Suggestions: Let cool for 10 minutes before slicing and serving.
7. Directions: & Cooking Tips: You'll also top the brownies with chopped walnuts.

Nutrition: Calories 68 Fat 6.1 g Carbohydrates 1.2 g

Sugar 0.3 g Protein 3 g Cholesterol 0 mg

Sugar 0.3 g Protein 3 g Cholesterol 0 mg

Easy Mug Brownie

Preparation Time:5 minutes

Cooking Time: 10 minutes

Servings:1

Ingredients:

- 1scoop chocolate protein powder
- 1tbsp cocoa powder
- 1/2 tsp baking powder
- 1/4 cup unsweetened almond milk

Directions:

1. Add baking powder, protein powder, and cocoa powder in a mug and mix well.
2. Add milk in a mug and stir well.
3. Place the mug in the air fryer and cook at 390 F for 10 minutes.
4. Serve and enjoy.

Nutrition: Calories 68 Fat 6.1 g Carbohydrates 1.2 g Sugar 0.3 g Protein 3 g Cholesterol 0 mg

Brownie Bites

Preparation Time:10 minutes

Cooking Time: 12 minutes

Servings:16

Ingredients:

- ¾ cup almond flour
- ½ tsp vanilla
- 2 eggs
- ½ cup unsweetened cocoa powder
- ¾ cup swerve
- 4 tbsp butter, melted Pinch of salt
- Directions:
- Preheat the air fryer to 325 F.
- In a bowl, whisk together butter, vanilla, eggs, cocoa powder, sweetener, and salt.
- Add almond flour and stir to combine.
- Pour batter into the mini silicone molds and place into the air fryer.
- Cook for 12 minutes or until done.
- Serve and enjoy.

Nutrition: Calories: 181 protein: 3 g. Fat: 98 g. Carbs: 42 g.

Yummy Brownies

Preparation Time:10 minutes

Cooking Time: 10 minutes

Servings:4

Ingredients:

- 2tbsp cocoa powder
- 1/4 tsp baking powder
- 1/2 tsp baking soda
- 2tbsp unsweetened applesauce
- 1tsp liquid stevia
- 1tbsp coconut oil, melted
- 3tbsp almond flour
- 1/2 tsp vanilla
- 1tbsp unsweetened almond milk
- 1/2 cup almond butter
- 1/4 tsp sea salt

Directions:

1. Preheat the air fryer to 350 F.
2. Grease air fryer baking dish with cooking spray and set aside.
3. In a small bowl, mix together almond flour, baking soda, cocoa powder, baking powder, and salt. Set aside.

4. In a small bowl, add coconut oil and almond butter and microwave until melted.

5. Add sweetener, vanilla, almond milk, and applesauce in the coconut oil mixture and stir well.

6. Add dry Ingredients: to the wet ingredients and stir to combine.

7. Pour batter into dish and place into the air fryer and cook for 10 minutes.

8. Slice and serve.

Nutrition: Calories: 185 protein: 4 g. Fat: 88 g. Carbs: 32 g.

Almond Bars

Preparation Time:10 minutes

Cooking Time: 35 minutes

Servings:12

Ingredients:

- 2 eggs, lightly beaten
- 1cup erythritol
- ½ tsp vanilla
- ¼ cup water
- ½ cup butter, softened
- ¾ cup cherries, pitted 1 ½ cup almond flour
- 1tbsp xanthan gum
- ½tsp salt

Directions:

1. In a bowl, mix together almond flour, erythritol, eggs, vanilla, butter, and salt until dough is formed.
2. Press dough in air fryer baking dish.
3. Place in the air fryer and cook at 375 F for 10 minutes.
4. Meanwhile, mix together cherries, xanthan gum, and water.

5. Pour cherry mixture over cooked dough and
cook for 25 minutes more.

6. Slice and serve.

Nutrition: Calories: 181 protein: 3 g. Fat: 98 g. Carbs: 42 g.

Chocolate Vanilla Bars

Preparation Time:10 Minutes

Cooking Time: 7 Minutes

Servings: 12

Ingredients:

- cup sugar free and vegan chocolate chips
- 2tablespoons coconut butter
- 2/3 cup coconut cream
- tablespoons stevia
- ¼ teaspoon vanilla extract

Directions:

1. Put the cream in a bowl, add stevia, butter and chocolate chips and stir
2. Leave aside for 5 minutes, stir well and mix the vanilla.
3. Transfer the mix into a lined baking sheet, introduce in your air fryer and cook at 356 degrees F for 7 minutes.
4. Leave the mix aside to cool down, slice and serve. Enjoy!

Nutrition: Calories: 120 Protein: 1 g. Fat: 5 g. Carbs: 6 g.

Raspberry Bars

Preparation Time:10 Minutes

Cooking Time: 6 Minutes

Servings: 12

Ingredients:

- 1/2 cup coconut butter, melted
- 1/2 cup coconut oil
- 1/2 cup raspberries, dried
- ¼ cup swerve
- 1/2 cup coconut, shredded

Directions:

1. In your food processor, blend dried berries very well.
2. In a bowl that fits your air fryer, mix oil with butter, swerve, coconut and raspberries, toss well, introduce in the fryer and cook at 320 degrees F for 6 minutes.
3. Spread this on a lined baking sheet, keep in the fridge for an hour, slice and serve.
4. Enjoy!

Nutrition: Calories: 164 Protein: 2 g. Fat: 22 g. Carbs: 4 g.

Oat Chocolate Cookies

Preparation Time:10 Minutes

Cooking Time: 20 Minutes

Servings: 8

Ingredients:

- cup unsalted butter, at room temperature
- cup dark brown sugar
- ½ cup granulated sugar
- large eggs
- tablespoon vanilla extract
- Pinch salt
- cups old-fashioned rolled oats
- 1½ cups all-purpose flour
- 1 teaspoon baking powder
- 1 teaspoon baking soda
- 2 cups chocolate chips

Directions:

1. Stir together the butter, granulated sugar, and brown sugar in a large mixing bowl until smooth and light in color.
2. Crack the eggs into the bowl, one at a Time, mixing after each addition. Stir in the vanilla and salt.

3. Mix together the oats, flour, baking soda, and baking powder in a separate bowl. Add the mixture to the butter mixture and stir until mixed. Stir in the chocolate chips.

4. Spread the dough onto the sheet pan in an even layer.

5. Place the basket on the bake position.

6. Select bake, set temperature to 350ºf (180ºc), and set Time to 20 minutes.

7. After 15 minutes, check the cookie, rotating the pan if the crust is not browning evenly. Continue cooking for a total of 18 to 20 minutes or until golden brown.

8. When cooking is complete, remove the pan from the air fryer grill and allow to cool completely before slicing and serving.

Nutrition: Calories: 184 Protein: 9 g. Fat: 6 g. Carbs: 24 g.

Italian Cookies

Preparation Time:15 minutes

Cooking Time: 18 Minutes.

Servings: 4

Ingredients:

- 4 cups flour
- cup butter
- 6 eggs
- 1 tsp. vanilla extract
- 1-1/2 cup sugar
- 1/4 tsp. salt

Instructions:

1. Beat the eggs until thick. Mix in melted butter.
2. Mix the remaining Ingredients: to make the batter.
3. Preheat the Power XL Air Fryer Grill to 200 0 C or 400 0 F.
4. Bake the batter in a waffle pan for 15-18 minutes.

Nutrition: Calories: 154 Protein: 8 g. Fat: 4 g. Carbs: 14 g.

Easy Coconut Cookies with Pecans

Preparation Time:10 minutes

Cooking Time: 25 minutes

Serves 10

Ingredients:

- 1/2cups coconut flour
- 1/2cups extra-fine almond flour
- 1/2teaspoon baking powder
- 11/3 teaspoon baking soda
- eggs plus an egg yolk, beaten
- 3/4cup coconut oil, at room temperature
- 1 cup unsalted pecan nuts, roughly chopped
- 3/4cup monk fruit
- 1/3teaspoon freshly grated nutmeg
- 1/3teaspoon ground cloves
- 1/2teaspoon pure vanilla extract
- 1/2teaspoon pure coconut extract
- 1/3teaspoon fine sea salt

Directions:

1. Line the air fry basket with parchment paper.

2. Mix the coconut flour, almond flour, baking soda, and baking powder in a large mixing bowl.
3. In another mixing bowl, stir together the coconut oil and eggs. Add the wet mixture to the dry mixture.
4. Mix in the remaining ingredients and stir until a soft dough form.
5. Drop about 2 tablespoons of dough on the parchment paper for each cookie and flatten each biscuit until it's 1 inch thick.
6. Place the basket on the bake position.
7. Select Bake, set temperature to 370ºF (188ºC), and set Time to 25 minutes.
8. When cooking is complete, the cookies should be golden and firm to the touch.
9. Remove from the air fryer grill to a plate. Let the cookies cool to room temperature and serve.

Nutrition: Calories: 237kcal, Carbs: 42g, Protein: 30g, Fat: 15g.

Coffee Cookies

Preparation Time:10 minutes

Cooking Time: 15 minutes

Servings:12

Ingredients:

- 1cup almond flour
- 2eggs, lightly beaten
- 2tsp baking powder
- ½tbsp cinnamon
- ¼cup erythritol
- ¼ cup brewed espresso
- ½ cup ghee, melted

Directions:

1. Add all Ingredients into the bowl and mix until well combined.
2. Place cookie sheet into the air fryer basket.
3. Make small cookies from mixture and place into the air fryer basket on cookie sheet.
4. Cook at 350 F for 15 minutes.
5. Serve and enjoy.

Nutrition: Calories: 184 Protein: 2 g. Fat: 12 g. Carbs: 3 g.

Choco Chips Cookies

Preparation Time:10 minutes

Cooking Time: 15 minutes

Servings:4

Ingredients:

- egg
- tbsp butter
- tsp vanilla
- ¼ tsp baking powder
- tbsp macadamia nuts, crushed
- 1 cup almond flour
- 2 tbsp unsweetened chocolate chips
- Pinch of salt

Directions:

1. In a bowl, beat egg using a hand mixer.
2. Add almond flour, butter, vanilla, baking powder, and salt and stir well.
3. Add Chocó chips and macadamia nuts and mix until dough is formed.
4. Preheat the air fryer to 360 F.
5. Make cookies from dough and place into the air fryer and cook for 15 minutes.
6. Serve and enjoy.

Nutrition: Calories: 194 Protein: 4 g. Fat: 22 g. Carbs: 3 g.

Peanut Butter Cookies

Preparation Time:5 minutes

Cooking Time: 12 minutes

Servings:15

Ingredients:

- egg
- ¼ cup erythritol
- 1cup peanut butter

Directions:

1. Preheat the air fryer to 325 F.
2. Add all Ingredients into the bowl and mix until well combined.
3. Make cookies from mixture and place into the air fryer and cook for 12 minutes.
4. Serve and enjoy.

Nutrition: Calories: 184 Protein: 2 g. Fat: 12 g. Carbs: 3 g.

Almond Pumpkin Cookies

Preparation Time:10 minutes

Cooking Time: 8 minutes

Servings:8

Ingredients:

- ¼ cup almond flour
- ½ cup pumpkin puree
- 3 tbsp swerve
- ½ tsp baking soda
- 1tbsp coconut flakes
- ½ tsp cinnamon Pinch of salt

Directions:

1. Preheat the air fryer to 360 F.
2. Add all Ingredients into the bowl and mix until well combined.
3. Spray air fryer basket with cooking spray.
4. Make cookies from bowl mixture and place into the air fryer and cook for 8 minutes.
5. Serve and enjoy.

Nutrition: Calories: 184 Protein: 2 g. Fat: 12 g. Carbs: 3 g.

Coconut Sunflower Cookies

Preparation Time:10 minutes

Cooking Time: 10 minutes

Servings:8

Ingredients:

- 5 oz sunflower seed butter
- 6 tbsp coconut flour
- tsp vanilla
- ¼ tsp olive oil
- tbsp swerve
- Pinch of salt

Directions:

1. Add all Ingredients into the bowl and mix until dough is formed.
2. Preheat the air fryer to 360 F.
3. Make cookies from mixture and place into the air fryer and cook for 10 minutes.
4. Serve and enjoy.

Nutrition: Calories: 184 Protein: 2 g. Fat: 12 g. Carbs: 3 g.

Cheese Butter Cookies

Preparation Time:10 minutes

Cooking Time: 12 minutes

Servings:8

Ingredients:

- 2 eggs
- 5 tbsp butter, melted
- 1/3 cup sour cream
- 1/3 cup mozzarella cheese, shredded
- 1/4 cup almond flour
- 1/2 tsp baking powder
- 1/2 tsp salt

Directions:

1. Preheat the air fryer to 370 F.
2. Add all Ingredients into a large bowl and mix using a hand mixer.
3. Spoon batter into the mini silicone muffin molds and place into the air fryer and cook for 12 minutes.
4. Serve and enjoy.

Nutrition: Calories: 214kcal, Carbs: 36g, Protein: 0.4g, Fat: 0.9g.

Vanilla Coconut Cheese Cookies

Preparation Time:10 minutes

Cooking Time: 12 minutes

Servings:15

Ingredients:

- egg
- 1/2 tsp baking powder
- tsp vanilla
- 1/2 cup swerve
- 1/2 cup butter, softened
- tbsp cream cheese, softened
- 1/2 cup coconut flour Pinch of salt

Directions:

1. In a bowl, beat together butter, sweetener, and cream cheese.
2. Add egg and vanilla and beat until smooth and creamy.
3. Add coconut flour, salt, and baking powder and beat until combined. Cover and place in the fridge for 1 hour.
4. Preheat the air fryer to 325 F.

5. Make cookies from dough and place into the air fryer and cook for 12 minutes.

6. Serve and enjoy.

Nutrition: Calories: 224kcal, Carbs: 46g, Protein: 1.4g, Fat: 0.9g.

Pumpkin Cookies

Preparation Time:10 minutes

Cooking Time: 20 minutes

Servings:27

Ingredients:

- egg
- cups almond flour
- 1/2 tsp baking powder
- 1 tsp vanilla
- 1/2 cup butter
- 15 drops liquid stevia
- 1/2 tsp pumpkin pie spice
- 1/2 cup pumpkin puree

Directions:

1. Preheat the air fryer to 280 F.
2. In a large bowl, add all ingredients and mix until well combined.
3. Make cookies from mixture and place into the air fryer and cook for 20 minutes.
4. Serve and enjoy.

Nutrition: Calories: 214kcal, Carbs: 36g, Protein: 0.4g, Fat: 0.9g.

Chia Chocolate Cookies

Preparation Time:5 minutes

Cooking Time: 8 minutes

Servings:20

Ingredients:

- 2 1/2 tbsp ground chia
- 2 tbsp chocolate protein powder
- cup sunflower seed butter
- 1 cup almond flour

Directions:

1. Preheat the air fryer to 325 F.
2. In a large bowl, add all ingredients and mix until combined.
3. Make cookies from bowl mixture and place into the air fryer and cook for 8 minutes.
4. Serve and enjoy.

Nutrition: Calories: 214kcal, Carbs: 36g, Protein: 0.4g, Fat: 0.9g.

Cinnamon Ginger Cookies

Preparation Time:10 minutes

Cooking Time: 12 minutes

Servings:8

Ingredients:

- egg
- 1/2 tsp vanilla
- 1/8 tsp ground cloves
- 1 tsp baking powder
- 3/4 cup erythritol
- 2/4 cup butter, melted
- 1 1/2 cups almond flour
- 1/4 tsp ground nutmeg
- 1/4 tsp ground cinnamon
- 1/2 tsp ground ginger Pinch of salt

Instructions:

1. In a large bowl, mix together all dry ingredients.
2. In a separate bowl, mix together all wet ingredients.
3. Add dry Ingredients: to the wet ingredients and mix until dough is formed. Cover and place in the fridge for 30 minutes.

4. Preheat the air fryer to 325 F.

5. Make cookies from dough and place into the air fryer and cook for 12 minutes.

Nutrition : Calories: 181 protein: 3 g. Fat: 98 g. Carbs: 42 g.

Lasagna Toast

Preparation Time:10 minutes

Cooking Time: 20 minutes

Servings: 4

Ingredients:

- 4 slices bread
- 4 cherry tomatoes, chopped
- small zucchini, chopped
- 1/2 cup cheddar cheese
- 1/2 cup mozzarella cheese
- 1 tbsp. olive oil
- 1 clove garlic

Directions:

1. Preheat the Power XL Air Fryer Grill to 2000C or 4000F.
2. Mix the veggies, spices, cheese, and oil in a bowl.
3. Spread the mixture all over the bread and top with another bread.
4. Toast it for 5 minutes.

Nutrition : Calories: 250kcal, Carbs: 16g, Protein: 35g, Fat: 9g.

Lamb Chops

Preparation Time:10 minutes

Cooking Time: 30 minutes

Servings: 4

Ingredients:

- 700gm lamb chops
- 1/3 cup olive oil
- tbsp. garlic, minced
- 1/2 tbsp. oregano
- tbsp. BBQ sauce
- tbsp. soy sauce
- Salt & pepper
- tbsp. lemon juice

Directions:

1. Preheat the Power XL Air Fryer Grill to 2000C or 4000F.
2. Mix all the ingredients in a pan.
3. Marinate the chops for 20 minutes with the mixture. Bake it in the Power XL Air Fryer Grill for 30 minutes Let it for 5 minutes before serving.

Nutrition: Calories: 294kcal, Protein: 25g, Fat: 21g.

Ham Avocado Toast

Preparation Time:5 minutes

Cooking Time: 5 minutes

Servings: 2

Ingredients:

- 2 wheat bread, sliced
- 4 slices deli ham - 1 ripe avocado
- 1/2 cup shredded cheese

Directions:

1. Toast the bread in the Power XL Air Fryer Grill until golden.
2. Mash the avocado and spread it on the bread along with two slices of ham. Evenly sprinkle the shredded cheese on top.
3. Bake until the cheese melts.

Nutrition: Calories: 155kcal, Carbs: 9g, Protein: 19g, Fat: 9g.

Baked Chicken Stew

Preparation Time:10 minutes

Cooking Time: 25 minutes

Servings: 2

Ingredients:

- cup boneless chicken, cut
- 1 large potato and 1 carrot, cut
- 1 stalk celery
- 1/2 tbsp. thyme
- 1 tbsp. flour
- 1 bay leaf
- 1 cup chicken stock
- Salt & pepper
- Cilantro, chopped

Directions:

1. Add 2 tbsp. water in the flour to make a slurry.
2. Mix all the ingredients in a bowl.
3. Cook it in the Power XL Air Fryer Grill with a foil lining.
4. Serve with fresh cilantro on top.

Nutrition: Calories: 237kcal, Carbs: 42g, Protein: 30g, Fat: 15g.

Tuna Melt Toastie

Preparation Time:5 minutes

Cooking Time: 10 minutes

Servings: 2

Ingredients:

- 150gm canned tuna
- 1/2 cup cilantro, chopped
- 2 slices wheat bread
- 3 tbsp. mayonnaise
- 50g mozzarella, grated
- Paprika.

Directions:

1. Preheat the Power XL Air Fryer Grill to 1500C or 3000F.
2. Mix all the ingredients except for bread.
3. Spread the tuna mixture on the bread and put the grated cheese on top.
4. Bake until the cheese melts.

Nutrition: Calories: 613kcal, Carbs: 10g, Protein: 35g, Fat: 40g.

Pizza Toast

Preparation Time:5 minutes

Cooking Time: 5 minutes

Servings: 2

Ingredients:

- 4 slices bread.
- 1/2 cup grated mozzarella.
- Pepperoni
- 1/2 tbsp. Italian herbs.
- 1/2 cup marinara sauce

Directions:

1. Spread marinara and grated cheese on the bread.
2. Put pepperoni and sprinkle some oregano.
3. Grill it in the preheated Power XL Air Fryer Grill for 5 minutes.

Nutrition: Calories: 175kcal, Carbs: 20g, Protein: 9g, Fat: 7g.

Baked Meatloaf

Preparation Time:20 minutes

Cooking Time: 40 minutes

Servings: 4

Ingredients:

- lb. ground beef
- onion, chopped
- 1/2 cup tomato, diced
- 1 tbsp. Italian herbs
- 1 tbsp. paprika
- 1 egg
- Salt & pepper
- 1/2 tbsp. garlic, minced
- tbsp. olive oil

Directions:

1. Preheat the Power XL Air Fryer Grill to 2320C or 4500F.
2. Combine all the ingredients in a bowl.
3. Grease a loaf pan with olive oil and put the mixture in it.
4. Bake it for 40 minutes.

Nutrition: Calories: 195kcal, Protein: 56g, Fat: 15g.

Strawberry Ricotta Toast

Preparation Time:5 minutes

Cooking Time: 5 minutes

Servings: 4

Ingredients:

- 2 slices of wheat bread
- 5 strawberries, chopped
- 100gm ricotta cheese
- tbsp. ground cinnamon
- eggs
- tbsp. pistachios
- Honey

Directions:

1. Whisk eggs with cinnamon in a bowl.
2. Soak the bread slices in the egg mixture.
3. Toast the bread in the preheated Power XL Air Fryer Grill.
4. Spread ricotta, strawberries, and pistachios on the freshly toasted bread.
5. Drizzle some honey on top.

Nutrition: Calories: 195kcal, Carbs: 10g, Protein: 15g, Fat: 4g.

Mediterranean Baked Fish

Preparation Time:10 minutes

Cooking Time: 10 minutes

Servings: 4

Ingredients:

- 4 white boneless fish fillets
- large onion, diced
- tomato, diced
- 1/2 tbsp. paprika
- 1/2 tbsp. cumin powder
- 1/2 tbsp. coriander powder
- 1 clove garlic, minced
- tbsp. olive oil
- 1/3 cup lime juice
- 1/2 cup of water

Directions:

1. Mix all the ingredients and marinate the fillets for 10 minutes.
2. Bake it in the Power XL Air Fryer Grill for 10 minutes.
3. Serve with fresh cilantro on top.

Nutrition: Calories: 170kcal, Protein: 14g, Fat: 35g.

Baked Cinnamon Apple

Preparation Time:5 minutes

Cooking Time: 10 minutes

Servings: 3

Ingredients:

- 3 apples, cut
- 1/2 tbsp. ground cinnamon
- 1/2 tbsp. vanilla
- tbsp. brown sugar

Directions:

1. Preheat the Power XL Air Fryer Grill to 1200C or 2500F.
2. Coat the apples with cinnamon, sugar, and vanilla.
3. Bake for 10 minutes. Serve with ice cream.

Nutrition: Calories: 214kcal, Carbs: 36g, Protein: 0.4g, Fat: 0.9g.

Maple-Glazed Sausages and Figs

Preparation Time: 30 minutes

Cooking Time: 9 minutes |

Servings: 2

Ingredients:

- 2 tbsp. maple syrup
- 2 tbsp. balsamic vinegar
- 2 packages of (12 ounces each) fully cooked chicken, cooked garlic sausages
- 8 fully ripe fresh figs, cut lengthwise
- 1/2 large sweet onion, minced
- 1-1/2 lbs. Swiss chard, with sliced stems, minced leaves
- 2 tsp. olive oil
- Salt and pepper

Directions:

1. Preheat the Power XL Air Fryer Grill to 2320C or 4500F, mix syrup with 1 tbsp. vinegar in a tiny bowl. Put sausages with figs on a one-layer foil-lined oven tray.
2. Roast for 8-10 minutes by grazing the syrup mix throughout the cooking.

3. Cook the onions in the Power XL Air Fryer Grill in a bowl with plastic wrap for 9 minutes.
4. Mix oil and seasoning with 1 tsp. vinegar. Serve the chards with figs and sausages.

Nutrition: Calories: 450kcal, Carbs: 42g, Protein: 34g, Fat: 17g.

Pumpkin Spice Bagels

Preparation Time: 10 minutes

Cooking Time: 25 minutes

Servings: 1

Ingredients:

- egg
- 1 cup flour
- 1/2 tsp. Pumpkin spice
- 1/2 cup Greek yogurt

Directions:

1. Create a dough with flour, pie spice, yogurt, and pumpkin in a stand mixer.
2. Shape the dough into a few ropes and make bagels.
3. Apply egg and water mixture over the bagels.
4. Preheat the powerxl air fryer grill to 190 0 c or 375 0 f and bake for 20-25 minutes.

Nutrition: Calories: 154 kcal Carbs: 9g Fat: 2.5g Protein: 8.6g

Southwestern Waffles

Preparation Time: 5 minutes

Cooking Time: 7minutes.

Servings: 1

Ingredients:

- egg, fried
- 1/4 avocado, chopped
- 1 frozen waffle
- 1 tbsp. Salsa

Directions:

1. Preheat the powerxl air fryer grill to 200 0 c or 400 0 f.
2. Bake the waffles for 5-7 minutes.
3. Add avocado, fried eggs, and fresh salsa as toppings.

Nutrition: Calories: 170 Carbs: 8 g Fat: 6 g Protein: 16 g

Wild Blueberry Bagels

Preparation Time: 5 minutes

Cooking Time: 5minutes.

Servings: 1

Ingredients:

- bagel
- tbsp. low-fat cream cheese
- tbsp. frozen wild blueberries
- 1/4 tsp. cinnamon

Directions:

1. Preheat the Power XL Air Fryer Grill to 190 0 C or 375 0 F
2. Toast the bagel for 3-5 minutes.
3. Spread cream cheese, add blueberry toppings, and cinnamon.

Nutrition: Calories: 145kcal, Carbs: 26g, Protein: 17.18g, Fat: 18g.

Brown Sugar Bacon Waffles

Preparation Time: 10 minutes

Cooking Time: 15 Minutes.

Servings: 7

Ingredients:

- 7 slices bacon
- 3 cups flour
- tbsp. baking powder
- 1 tsp. baking soda and salt
- 1/2 cup brown sugar
- 4 eggs
- tsp. vanilla extract
- 2/3 cup grapeseed oil
- cups buttermilk

Directions:

1. Mix all dry ingredients and then wet Ingredients: to make the batter.
2. Preheat the Power XL Air Fryer Grill to 180 0 C or 350 0 F
3. Grease the waffle pan, pour the mix and bake for 15 minutes.

Nutrition: Calories: 245kcal, Carbs: 28g, Protein:

16.18g, Fat: 18.53g.

Buttermilk Waffles

Preparation Time:10 minutes

Cooking Time: 4 Minutes.

Servings: 5

Ingredient:

- 2 eggs
- 2 cups of flour
- 2 tsp. sugar and vanilla extract
- tsp. salt and baking soda
- tsp. baking powder
- cups of buttermilk
- 1/2 cup of butter

Directions:

1. Whisk all the dry Ingredients: then the wet ingredients in a bowl.
2. Preheat the Power XL Air Fryer Grill at 1500C or 3000F and bake for 3-4 minutes.

Nutrition: Calories: 423 kcal, Carbs: 43g, Protein: 9g, Fat: 23g.

Simple Bagel

Preparation Time: 10 minutes

Cooking Time: 25 Minutes.

Servings: 4

Ingredients:

- cup of flour
- egg white, beaten
- tsp. salt
- tsp. baking powder
- 1 cup of yogurt.

Directions:

1. Add all the Ingredients: to form the dough.
2. Knead the dough until tacky.
3. Make small balls and roll them to give a shape.
4. Sprinkle toppings if required.
5. Preheat the Power XL Air Fryer Grill to 1900C or 3750F and bake for 20-25 minutes.

Nutrition: Calories: 152cal, Carbs: 26.5g, Protein: 10g, Fat: 0.3g.

Italian Waffle Cookies

Preparation Time:20 minutes

Cooking Time: 18 Minutes.

Servings: 4

Ingredients:

- 4 cups of flour
- cup of butter
- 6 eggs
- 1 tsp. vanilla extract
- 1-1/2 cup of sugar
- 1/4 tsp. salt

Directions:

1. Beat the eggs until thick. Mix in melted butter.
2. Mix the remaining Ingredients: to form the batter.
3. Preheat the Power XL Air Fryer Grill to 2000C or 4000F.
4. Bake the batter in a waffle pan for 15-18 minutes.

Nutrition: Calories: 132kcal, Carbs: 17g, Protein: 2g, Fat: 5g.

Strawberry Ricotta Waffles

Preparation Time: 10 minutes

Cooking Time: 15 Minutes.

Servings: 2

Ingredients:

- 2 cups of flour
- tsp. baking soda, 2tsp baking powder
- eggs
- tbsp. sugar
- 1/2 tsp. vanilla extract
- 2 cups of milk
- 1/4 cup of oil
- 1/2 cup of strawberries, sliced
- 1/4 cup of ricotta cheese
- 2 tsp. maple syrup

Directions:

1. Preheat the Power XL Air Fryer Grill to 2000C or 4000F
2. Whisk the dry and wet batter ingredients.
3. pour batter into the mold and bake for 12-15 minutes.
4. Mix ricotta and vanilla in a bowl. Top with the mixture, syrup, and strawberries.

Nutrition: Calories: 318cal, Carbs: 43.1g, Protein: 11.9g, Fat: 13.6g.

Pineapple Bagel Brulees

Preparation Time:15 minutes

Cooking Time: 10 Minutes.

Servings: 8

Ingredients:

- 4 thin bagels
- 4 tsp. brown sugar
- 3/4 cup of low-fat cream cheese
- 8 slices pineapples
- 3 tbsp. almonds, toasted

Directions:

1. Preheat the Power XL Air Fryer Grill at 2200C or 4250F.
2. Bake the pineapple slices with sugar sprinkled on top.
3. Toast bagels, and apply cheese, almonds, and baked pineapples.

Nutrition: Calories: 157cal, Carbs: 22.9g, Protein: 5.6g, Fat: 6.4g.

Golden Egg Bagels

Preparation Time:15 minutes

Cooking Time: 20 Minutes.

Servings: 8

Ingredients:

- 2 eggs
- 4 tsp. dry yeast
- 4-5 cup of all-purpose flour
- tbsp. canola oil and kosher salt
- 1-1/2 tbsp. sugar

Directions:

1. Whisk eggs, sugar, yeast, lukewarm, water, and oil. Add flour and salt to organize the dough.
2. Make an extended rope with the dough, locking both ends.
3. Preheat the Power XL Air Fryer Grill to 2000C or 4000F.
4. Boil bagels in sugar and salt for 45 seconds.
5. Drain bagels, brush with albumen and bake for 15-20 mins.

Nutrition: Calories: 164cal, Carbs: 28.4g, Protein: 6.6g, Fat: 2.1g.

Roasted Parsnip Sticks with Salted Caramel

Preparation Time:5 Minutes

Cooking Time: 25 Minutes

Servings: 4

Ingredients:

- 1-pound parsnip, trimmed, scrubbed, cut into sticks
- Two tablespoon avocado oil
- Two tablespoons granulated sugar
- Two tablespoons butter
- 1/4 teaspoon ground allspice

Directions:

1. Toss the parsnip with the avocado oil; bake in the preheated Air Fryer at 380 degrees F for 15 minutes, and occasionally shake the cooking basket to ensure even cooking.
2. Then, heat the sugar and one tablespoon of water in a small pan over medium heat. Cook until the sugar has dissolved; bring to a boil.
3. Keep swirling the pan around until the sugar reaches a rich caramel color. Pour in

2 tablespoons of cold water. Now, add the butter, allspice, and salt. The mixture should be runny.

4. Afterward, drizzle the salted caramel over the roasted parsnip sticks and enjoy!

Nutrition: Calories 213 Fat 11g Carbs 24g Protein 4g Sugar 3g

Smoky BBQ Roasted Almonds

Preparation Time:5 Minutes

Cooking Time: 6 Minutes

Servings: 4

Ingredients:

- cup of raw almonds
- Two teaspoons coconut oil
- One teaspoon chili powder
- ¼ teaspoon cumin
- ¼ teaspoon smoked paprika

Directions:

1. In a large bowl, toss all fixings until almonds are evenly coated with oil and spices. Place almonds into the air fryer basket.
2. Regulate the temperature to 320°F and set the Timer for 6 minutes.
3. Toss the fryer basket midway through the cooking Time.
4. Allow cooling completely.

Nutrition: Calories: 182 Protein: 6.2 g Fiber: 3.3 g

Net carbohydrates: 3.3 g Fat: 16.3 g Sodium: 19 mg

Carbohydrates: 6.6 g Sugar: 1.1 g

Ranch Roasted Almonds

Preparation Time:5 Minutes

Cooking Time: 6 Minutes

Servings: 8

Ingredients:

- 2 cups of raw almonds
- Two tablespoons unsalted butter, melted
- ½ (1-ounce) ranch dressing mix packet

Directions:

1. In a large container, chuck almonds in butter to lightly coat. Sprinkle ranch mix over almonds and toss. Place almonds into the air fryer basket.
2. Alter the temperature to 320°F and set the Timer for 6 minutes.
3. Shake the basket two- or three Times during cooking.
4. Let cool at least 20 minutes. Almonds will be soft but become crunchier during cooling—stock in an airtight vessel for up to 3 days.

Nutrition: Calories: 190 Protein: 6.0 g Fiber: 3.0 g

Net carbohydrates: 4.0 g Fat: 16.7 g Sodium: 133

mg Carbohydrates: 7.0 g Sugar: 1.0 g

Roasted Ravioli

Preparation Time:10 Minutes

Cooking Time: 15 Minutes

Servings: 4

Ingredients:

- package ravioli, frozen
- cup breadcrumbs
- 1/2 cup parmesan cheese
- tbs. Italian seasoning
- tbs. garlic powder
- eggs, beaten
- Cooking spray

Directions:

1. Mix breadcrumbs with garlic powder, cheese, and Italian seasoning in a bowl.
2. Whisk eggs in another bowl. Dip each ravioli in eggs first then coat them with crumbs mixture.
3. Place the ravioli in the Air Fryer basket. Set the Air Fryer basket inside the Air Fryer toaster oven and close the lid. Select the Air Fry mode at 360°F temperature for 15

minutes. Flip the ravioli after 8 minutes and resume cooking.

4. Serve warm.

Nutrition: Calories: 124 Cal Protein: 4.5 g Carbs: 27.5 g Fat: 3.5 g

Roasted Eggplant Fries

Preparation Time:10 Minutes

Cooking Time: 20 Minutes

Servings: 4

Ingredients:

- 1/2 cup panko breadcrumbs
- 1/2 tsp. salt
- eggplant, peeled and sliced
- 1 cup egg, whisked

Directions:

1. Toss the breadcrumbs with salt in a tray. Dip the eggplant in the whisked egg and coat with the crumb's mixture.
2. Place the eggplant slices in the Air Fryer basket.
3. Set the Air Fryer basket inside the Air Fryer toaster oven and close the lid. Select the Air Fry mode at 400°F temperature for 20 minutes. Flip the slices after 10 minutes then resume cooking. Serve warm.

Nutrition: Calories: 110 Cal Protein: 5 g Carbs: 12.8 g Fat: 11.9 g

Roasted Stuffed Eggplants

Preparation Time:10 Minutes

Cooking Time: 38 Minutes

Servings: 4

Ingredients:

- 2 eggplants, cut in half lengthwise
- 1/2 cup shredded cheddar cheese
- 1/2 can (7.5 oz.) chili without beans
- 2 tsp. kosher salt
- 2 tbsp. cooked bacon bits
- 2 tbsp. sour cream
- Fresh scallions, thinly sliced

Directions:

1. Place the eggplants halves in the Air Fryer basket. Set the basket inside the Air Fryer toaster oven and close the lid. Select the Air Fry mode at 390°F temperature for 35 minutes.

2. Top each eggplant half with chili, cheese, and salt. Place the halves in a baking pan and return to the oven. Select the Broil mode at 375°F temperature for 3 minutes.

3. Garnish with bacon bits, sour cream, and scallions. Serve.

Nutrition: Calories: 113 Cal Protein: 9.2 g Carbs: 13 g Fat: 21 g

Roasted Bacon Poppers

Preparation Time:10 Minutes

Cooking Time: 15 Minutes

Servings: 4

Ingredients:

- 4 strips bacon, crispy cooked
- Dough:
- 2/3 cup water
- 3 tbsp. butter
- tbsp. bacon fat
- tsp. kosher salt
- 2/3 cup all-purpose flour
- eggs
- oz. Cheddar cheese, shredded
- 1/2 cup jalapeno peppers
- A pinch pepper
- A pinch black pepper

Directions:

1. Whisk butter with water and salt in a skillet over medium heat. Stir in flour, then stir cook for about 3 minutes. Transfer this flour to a bowl, then whisk in eggs and rest of the ingredients.

2. Fold in bacon and mix well. Wrap this dough in a plastic sheet and refrigerate for 30 minutes. Make small balls out of this dough.

3. Place these bacon balls in the Air Fryer basket. Set the basket inside the Air Fryer toaster oven and close the lid. Select the Air Fry mode at 390°F temperature for 15 minutes. Flip the balls after 7 minutes then resume cooking.

4. Serve warm.

Nutrition: Calories: 240 Cal Protein: 14.9 g Carbs: 7.1 g Fat: 22.5 g

Roasted Almonds

Preparation Time:5 minutes

Cooking Time: 8 minutes

Servings:8

Ingredients:

- 2 cups almonds
- 1/4 tsp pepper
- tsp paprika
- 1 tbsp garlic powder
- 1 tbsp soy sauce

Directions:

1. Add pepper, paprika, garlic powder, and soy sauce in a bowl and stir well.
2. Add almonds and stir to coat.
3. Spray air fryer basket with cooking spray.
4. Add almonds in air fryer basket and cook for 6-8 minutes at 320 F. Shake basket after every 2 minutes.
5. Serve and enjoy.

Nutrition: Calories 172 Fat 12.6 g Carbohydrates 15.7 g Sugar 7.6 g Protein 6 g Cholesterol 2 mg

Roasted Spaghetti Squash

Preparation Time 20 minutes

Cooking Time: 10 Minutes

Servings: 4

Ingredients:

- ripe squash
- Salt & pepper

Directions:

1. Preheat the Power XL Air Fryer Grill to 1500C or 3000F.
2. Prick the surface of the cleaned squash with a fork.
3. Roast it for 10 minutes.
4. Cut the roasted squash and scrape out the strands.
5. Sprinkle salt and pepper and serve.

Nutrition: Calories: 42kcal, Carbs: 3g, Protein: 1g, Fat: 0.5g,

Roasted Filet Mignon

Preparation Time 20 minutes

Cooking Time: 30 minutes

Servings: 2

Ingredients:

- 10 ounces filet mignon
- tbsp. Italian herbs, chopped
- Salt & pepper
- tbsp. olive oil

Directions:

1. Preheat the Power XL Air Fryer Grill to 2000C or 4000F.
2. Mix all the seasonings and oil, and rub the mixture on the steak.
3. Roast it for a half-hour.

Nutrition: Calories: 267kcal, Protein: 26g, Fat: 17g

Roasted Pears

Preparation Time 40 minutes

Cooking Time:20 minutes

Servings: 3

Ingredients:

- 3 semi-ripe pears
- 1/2 cup of icing sugar
- 2 tbsp. butter
- tbsp. ground cinnamon
- 3/4 cup of white wine

Directions:

1. Mix all the ingredients, apart from pears.
2. Prick the pears with a fork and let them soak in the wine mixture for a quarter-hour.
3. Roast in the preheated Power XL Air Fryer Grill for 20 minutes.

Nutrition: Calories: 103kcal, Carbs: 27g, Protein: 1g, Fat: 4g

Roasted Italian Sausage

Preparation Time 10 minutes

Cooking Time:20 minutes

Servings: 4

Ingredients:

- 4 Italian sausage
- large potato, chopped
- ounces mushroom, chopped
- 1tbsp Italian herbs
- tbsp. paprika
- Salt
- 1 clove garlic
- tbsp. olive oil

Directions:

1. Mix the seasonings and oil in a pan and coat the sausages and veggies.
2. Roast in the Power XL Air Fryer Grill for 20 minutes.

Nutrition: Calories: 81kcal, Carbs: 60g, Protein: 4.7g, Fat: 7g

Roasted Vegetable Pasta

Preparation Time 10 minutes

Cooking Time:20 minutes

Servings: 4

Ingredients:

- 10-ounce linguine pasta
- 1/2 cup of cilantro, chopped
- 5 cherry tomatoes, chopped
- zucchini, chopped
- 1/2 cup of marinara sauce
- Salt & pepper
- 1/2 cup of parmesan cheese
- tbsp. olive oil

Directions:

1. Preheat the Power XL Air Fryer Grill to 1500C or 3000F.
2. Stir in the veggies, pasta, and spices in a bowl with some water.
3. Roast for 20 minutes.
4. Sprinkle parmesan cheese on top.

Nutrition: Calories: 179kcal, carbs: 40g, Protein: 6.3g, Fat: 1.5g

Roasted Sweet Potato Tater Tots

Preparation Time: 10 Minutes

Cooking Time: 23 Minutes

Servings: 4

Ingredients:

- 2 sweet potatoes, peeled
- 1/2 tsp. Cajun seasoning
- Olive oil cooking spray
- Sea salt to taste

Directions:

1. Boil sweet potatoes in water for 15 minutes over medium-high heat.
2. Drain the sweet potatoes then allow them to cool.
3. Peel the boiled sweet potatoes and return them to the bowl.
4. Mash the potatoes and stir in salt and Cajun seasoning. Mix well and make small tater tots out of it.
5. Place the tater tots in the Air Fryer basket and spray them with cooking oil. Set the Air Fryer basket inside the Air Fryer toaster

oven and close the lid. Select the Air Fry
mode at 400°F temperature for 8 minutes.
Flip the tater tots and continue cooking for
another 8 minutes.

6. Serve fresh.

Nutrition: Calories: 184 Cal Protein: 9 g Carbs: 43 g
Fat: 17 g

Miso Glazed Salmon

Preparation time: 10 minutes

Cooking Time:5 minutes

Servings: 4

Ingredients:

- 4 salmon filets
- 1/4 cup miso
- 1/3 cup sugar
- tsp. soy sauce
- 1/3 cup sake
- tsp. vegetable oil

Directions:

1. Whisk all the ingredients, except for filets, in a bowl.
2. Marinate the filets with the mixture for 10 minutes.
3. Preheat the Power XL Air Fryer Grill to high and roast it for 5 minutes.

Nutrition: Calories: 331.8kcal, Carbs: 2gProtein: 34 g, Fat: 17.9 g.

Fireless S'mores

Preparation Time 5 minutes

Cooking Time:2minutes

Servings: 4

Ingredients:

- 8 graham crackers
- 4 marshmallows
- dark chocolate bar, chopped

Directions:

1. Put all the Ingredients: on top of the graham cracker and top with another cracker.
2. Roast it in the Power XL Air Fryer Grill for 2 minutes.

Nutrition: Calories: 87kcal, Carbs: 6g, Protein: 01g, Fat: 03 g.

Standing Rib Roast

This classic and comforting holiday meal is beyond any description.

Preparation time 30 minutes

Cooking Time:60 minutes

Servings: 8

Ingredients:

- 5 lb. rib-eye meat
- Salt & pepper
- tbsp. thyme
- 1 tbsp. rosemary
- 1 stick unsalted butter

Directions:

1. Preheat the Power XL Air Fryer Grill to 2300C or 4500F.
2. Mix the butter and dry ingredients in a bowl.
3. Rub the mixture on the rib and roast it for an hour in the preheated Power XL Air Fryer Grill.
4. Serve with fresh herbs on top.

Nutrition: Calories: 185kcal, Protein: 52.0 g, Fat: 48 g.

Air Roasted Steak

Preparation Time:5 minutes

Cooking Time: 15 minutes

Servings: 2

Ingredients:

- 2 rib-eye steaks, sliced 1-1/2- inch pieces
- 1/2 cup soy sauce
- 1/4 cup olive oil
- 4 teaspoons grill seasoning

Directions:

1. In a resealable bag, combine steaks, seasoning, olive oil and soy sauce; shake to coat well and let marinate for at least 2 hours.
2. Remove the meat from the bag and discard the marinade.
3. Add a splash of water to the air fryer toast oven pan and then preheat to 400 degrees.
4. Add the meat to the basket and air roast for 7 minutes.
5. Turn over the steak and air roast for another 8 minutes.

6. Turn off the air fry oven and let rest for at least 5 minutes before serving.

Nutrition: Calories: 652 kcal, Carbs: 7.5 g, Fat: 49.1g, Protein: 44 g.

Air Roasted Pork Ribs

Preparation Time:2-12 hours

Cooking Time: 15 minutes

Servings: 4

Ingredients:

- rack pork baby back ribs
- tbsp. oyster sauce
- tbsp. light soy sauce
- tsp. dark soy sauce
- 1 tbsp. mustard
- 1-1/2 tbsp. pure honey
- 5 cloves garlic, halved
- 1-inch fresh garlic, sliced
- For the sauce:
- 1 tbsp. soy sauce
- 1 tbsp. fish sauce
- tsp. toasted rice powder
- 1 tsp. sugar
- 2 tsp. red chili flakes
- Freshly squeezed juice of 1/2 a lemon
- 2 tsp. finely chopped cilantro
- 1 clove garlic, finely chopped

Directions:

1. Combine all the Ingredients: for the ribs, apart from the ribs, in a bowl to make the marinade.

2. Separate the ribs and pour the marinade over the ribs in a large bowl ensuring the ribs are well coated. Cover with cling wrap and marinate for a minimum of 2 hours. For best results, marinate overnight.

3. Set your air fry toaster oven to 360 degrees F,

4. Add the ribs, garlic and ginger pieces into the air fryer toast oven. Do not add the juices. Air roast for six minutes, shake well and cook for another 6 minutes.

5. As the ribs are cooking, make the dip by combining all the sauce Ingredients: then set aside in a small bowl.

6. Serve the ribs hot with the dipping sauce.

7. Enjoy!

Nutrition: Calories: 456 kcal, Carbs: 19.7 g, Fat: 15.2 g, Protein: 26.3 g.

Air Roasted Lamb

Preparation Time:5 minutes

Cooking Time: 1 hour

Servings: 4

Ingredients:

- 1-1/4 kg Leg of Lamb
- tablespoon olive oil
- A pinch of sea salt
- Pepper

Directions:

1. Season the leg of lamb with salt and pepper and place it in the fryer basket.
2. Air roast for 20 minutes at 360 degrees, turn the leg of lamb over and continue roasted for another 20 minutes.
3. Serve with roasted potatoes.

Nutrition: Calories: 639 kcal, Carbs: 10.8 g, Fat: 22.6 g, Protein: 102.6 g.

Asian Air Broiled Pork Chops

Preparation Time:15 minutes

Cooking Time: 20 minutes

Servings: 4

Ingredients:

- 450g pork chops
- 3/4 cup corn/potato starch
- egg white
- 1/4 tsp. freshly ground black pepper
- 1/2 tsp. kosher salt
- For the stir fry:
- green onions, sliced
- jalapeno peppers, seeds removed and sliced
- 2 tbsp. peanut oil
- 1/4 tsp. freshly ground pepper and kosher salt to taste

Directions:

1. Brush or spray the basket of your air fryer toast oven with oil.

2. Next, whisk the egg, black pepper and salt until it gets frothy. Cut up the pork chops

and use a clean kitchen towel to pat the meat dry.

3. Toss the cutlets in the frothy egg mixture until evenly coated. Cover and marinate for 30 minutes.

4. Place the pork chops in a separate bowl and pour in the corn/ potato starch ensuring each culet is thoroughly dredged. Shake off the excess corn/ potato starch and arrange the pork chops on the basket.

5. Set the air fry toaster oven on air roast at 360 degrees F and cook for 9 minutes, shaking the basket after every 2-3 minutes and spraying or brushing the cutlets with more oil if needed.

6. Turn to broil and cook for 6 more minutes or until the chops are crisp and done to desire.

7. Heat a wok or pan over high heat until extremely hot. Add all the stir fry ingredients and sauté for a minute.

8. Add your cooked pork chops and toss with the stir fry.

9. Cook for another minute ensuring the pork chops are evenly coated with the stir fry ingredients. Enjoy!

Nutrition: Calories: 398 kcal, Carbs: 16.1 g, Fat: 17.5 g, Protein: 21.1 g.